Renal Diet CookBook for Beginners

Essential Recipes for Kidney Health

Lorraine M. Smith

TABLE OF CONTENTS

INTRODUCTION

Sofia found herself at a crossroads in her life in the tranquil suburb of Willow Grove. With renal problems, she understood that a big adjustment in her lifestyle was necessary for her health. Sofia set out on a mission to take control over her well-being after becoming frustrated with the constraints imposed by her illness.

In her search for a better lifestyle, Sofia came upon the "Renal Diet Cookbook for Beginners." She enthusiastically dove into the pages of this gourmet book, drawn in by the promises of increased kidney function and overall well-being. The cookbook, created expressly for persons with kidney issues, promised a treasure trove of tasty and kidney-friendly recipes that will convert her meals into a source of food and healing.

Sofia began to change her eating habits after reading the cookbook. She ditched manufactured meals and excessive salt in favor of fresh, nutrient-dense cuisine customized to her renal health. The cookbook became her valued friend, leading her through the complexities of meal planning and assisting her in making intelligent food choices.

The simplicity of the recipes was one of the things that drew Sofia in. As a newcomer to renal diets, she enjoyed the simple directions and readily available products. The guidebook served as a culinary mentor, allowing Sofia to explore with tastes while adhering to her dietary constraints.

The Renal Diet Cookbook had a significant influence on Sofia's health. Her energy levels improved with time, and her renal function showed signs of stability. The meticulously crafted meals not only met her medical demands, but also her taste buds, demonstrating that a renal diet could be both healthy and delightful.

Aside from the physical benefits, Sofia found the cookbook to be a source of inspiration. It sparked her interest in cooking and inspired her to see her dietary constraints as an opportunity for creativity and self-care rather than a barrier. She developed a new joy for nutritious, home-cooked meals that nourished both her body and spirit.

Sofia's adventure with the Renal Diet Cookbook for Beginners was more than simply restoring her health; it was a life-changing event that changed her relationship with food. Sofia found herself on a path to holistic rehabilitation as she proceeded to explore the cookbook's numerous and wonderful dishes, guided by the wisdom of a cookbook that had become her ally in the search of a better, more vibrant existence.

CHAPTER 1.

RENTAL DIET BASICS:

Budget-Friendly Rental Diet Basics
- One-Pan Chicken and Veggie
Delight

INGREDIENTS:

- 4 boneless, skinless chicken breasts
- 1 pound baby potatoes, halved
- 2 cups baby carrots
- 1 broccoli crown, cut into florets
- 1 bell pepper, sliced
- 1 red onion, sliced
- 3 tablespoons olive oil
- 2 teaspoons garlic powder

- 1 teaspoon dried oregano
- 1 teaspoon paprika
- Salt and pepper to taste
- Fresh parsley for garnish (optional)

INSTRUCTIONS:

1. Preheat the oven to 400 degrees Fahrenheit (200 degrees Celsius).

2. Combine the halved baby potatoes, baby carrots, broccoli florets, sliced bell pepper, and red onion in a large mixing dish.

3. Season both sides of the chicken breasts with garlic powder, dried oregano, paprika, salt, and pepper on a cutting board.

4. In a large oven-safe skillet over medium-high heat, heat the olive oil.

5. Add the seasoned chicken breasts to the skillet once the oil is heated. Sear each side for 2-3 minutes, or until golden brown.

6. Push the cooked chicken breasts to the side of the skillet and add the mixed veggies, distributing them around the chicken.

7. Drizzle more olive oil over the veggies and season with salt and pepper to taste. Toss the veggies in the oil and spices to coat.

8. Bake for 20-25 minutes, or until the chicken reaches an internal temperature

of 165°F (74°C) and the veggies are cooked, in a preheated oven.

9. Remove the pan from the oven and set it aside for a few minutes to cool.

10. If desired, garnish with fresh parsley.

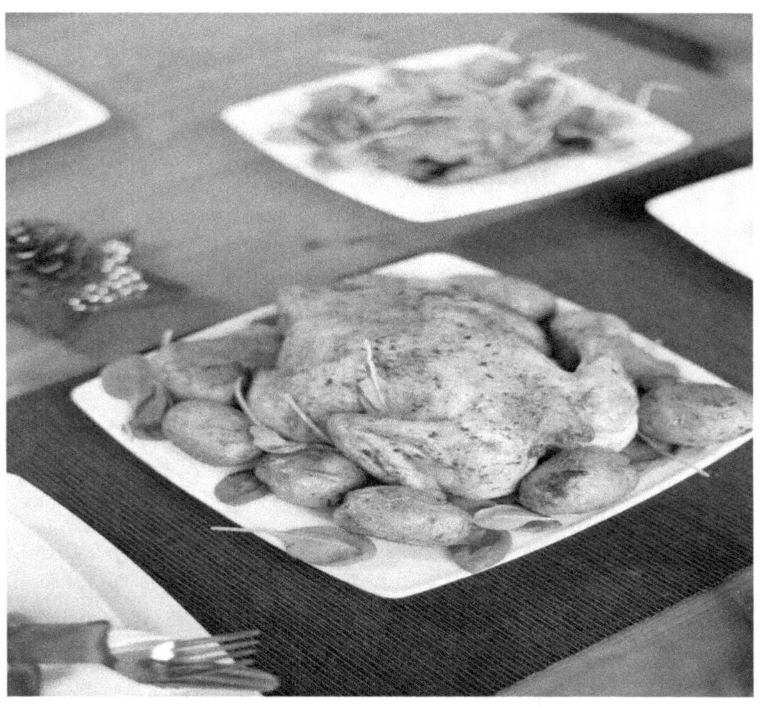

CHAPTER 2.

KEY NUTRIENTS FOR RENAL HEALTH:

Renal-Friendly Quinoa and Vegetable Bowl

INGREDIENTS:

- 1 cup quinoa, rinsed

- 2 cups low-sodium vegetable broth

- 1 tablespoon olive oil

- 1 medium onion, finely chopped

- 2 cloves garlic, minced

- 1 cup cherry tomatoes, halved

- 1 cup cucumber, diced

- 1 cup bell peppers (mix of colors), diced

- 1 cup zucchini, diced

- 1 cup cooked and shredded chicken (optional for added protein)

- 1/4 cup fresh parsley, chopped

- 2 tablespoons lemon juice

- Salt and pepper to taste

INSTRUCTIONS:

1. Combine quinoa and low-sodium vegetable broth in a medium saucepan. Bring to a boil, then lower to a low heat, cover, and cook for 15-20 minutes, or until the quinoa is tender and the liquid has been absorbed.

2. In a large pan over medium heat, heat the olive oil while the quinoa is cooking. Sauté the onion and garlic until softened and aromatic.

3. To the skillet, add chopped bell peppers, zucchini, and cucumber. Cook for 5-7 minutes, or until the veggies are cooked but still crisp.

4. If using chicken, combine the cooked and shredded chicken with the veggies in the skillet.

5. When the quinoa has finished cooking, fluff it with a fork and add it to the pan with the veggies and chicken. Combine all of the ingredients.

6. Combine the halved cherry tomatoes, fresh parsley, and lemon juice in a mixing bowl. Season to taste with salt and pepper. Toss the ingredients together carefully.

7. Remove the skillet from the heat and set aside for a few minutes to let the flavors to blend.

8. Warm the kidney-friendly quinoa and veggie dish. If required, adjust the seasoning.

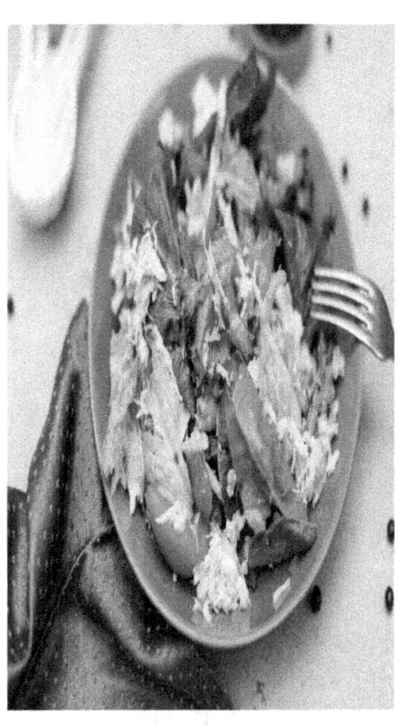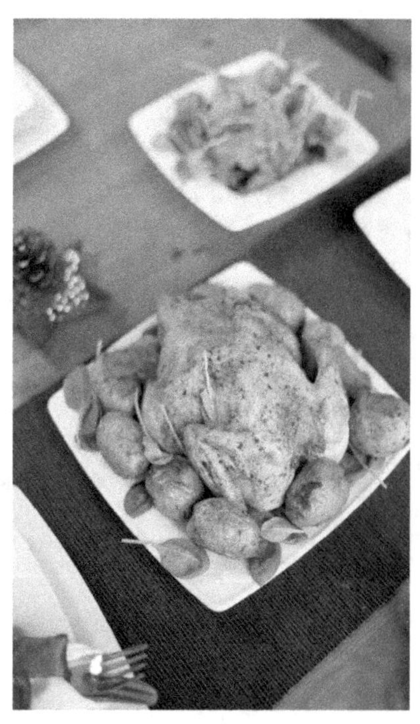

CHAPTER 3.

MEAL PLANNING FOR RENAL DIETS:

Renal-Friendly Chicken and Vegetable Stir-Fry with Brown Rice

INGREDIENTS:

- 1 cup brown rice, uncooked
- 2 cups water
- 2 tablespoons low-sodium soy sauce
- 1 tablespoon olive oil
- 1 pound boneless, skinless chicken breasts, thinly sliced
- 2 cloves garlic, minced

- 1 teaspoon fresh ginger, grated
- 1 cup broccoli florets
- 1 cup snap peas, trimmed
- 1 red bell pepper, thinly sliced
- 1 carrot, julienned
- 2 green onions, sliced
- 1 tablespoon rice vinegar
- 1 teaspoon sesame oil
- Sesame seeds for garnish (optional)

INSTRUCTIONS:

1. Cook brown rice according to package instructions, using 2 cups of water. Set aside.

2. In a small bowl, mix low-sodium soy sauce and set aside.

3. Heat olive oil in a large skillet or wok over medium-high heat.

4. Add sliced chicken and cook until browned and cooked through. Remove the chicken from the skillet and set aside.

5. In the same skillet, add minced garlic and grated ginger. Sauté for 1-2 minutes until fragrant.

6. Add broccoli florets, snap peas, red bell pepper, and julienned carrot to the skillet. Stir-fry for 3-4 minutes until the vegetables are tender-crisp.

7. Return the cooked chicken to the skillet and mix with the vegetables.

8. Pour the prepared soy sauce over the chicken and vegetables. Stir to combine and ensure even coating.

9. Drizzle rice vinegar and sesame oil over the stir-fry. Toss the ingredients to incorporate the flavors.

10. Add sliced green onions and cook for an additional 1-2 minutes.

11. Serve the renal-friendly chicken and vegetable stir-fry over the cooked brown rice.

12. Garnish with sesame seeds if desired.

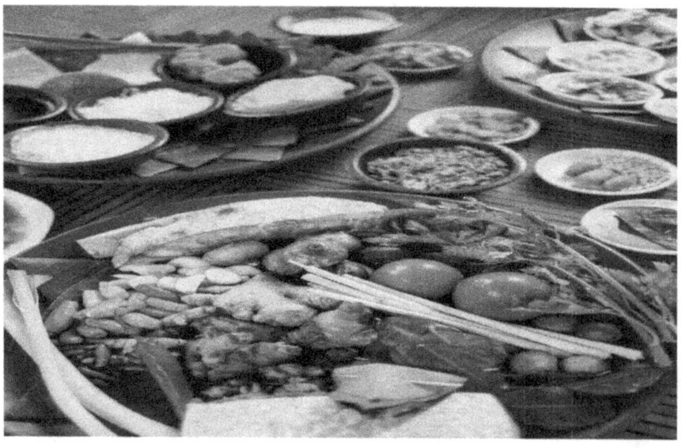

CHAPTER 4.

DELICIOUS AND NUTRIENT-RICH RECIPES:

Mediterranean Chickpea Salad

INGREDIENTS:

- 2 cans (15 oz each) chickpeas, drained and rinsed
- 1 cucumber, diced
- 1 cup cherry tomatoes, halved
- 1/2 red onion, finely chopped
- 1/2 cup Kalamata olives, sliced
- 1/2 cup crumbled feta cheese

- 1/4 cup fresh parsley, chopped
- 1/4 cup fresh mint, chopped
- 3 tablespoons extra-virgin olive oil
- 2 tablespoons red wine vinegar
- 1 teaspoon dried oregano
- Salt and pepper to taste
- Lemon wedges for serving (optional)

INSTRUCTIONS:

1. Combine chickpeas, diced cucumber, cherry tomatoes, chopped red onion, sliced Kalamata olives, crumbled feta cheese, fresh parsley, and fresh mint in a large mixing dish.

2. To make the dressing, mix together extra-virgin olive oil, red wine vinegar, dried oregano, salt, and pepper in a small bowl.

3. Toss the chickpea mixture with the dressing to coat all of the ingredients.

4. enable the salad to marinade for at least 30 minutes in the refrigerator to enable the flavors to mingle.

5. Give the salad one more toss before serving, and adjust the spice as required.

6. Serve the Mediterranean Chickpea Salad in bowls or on a tray, if preferred garnish ed with fresh herbs and lemon wedges.

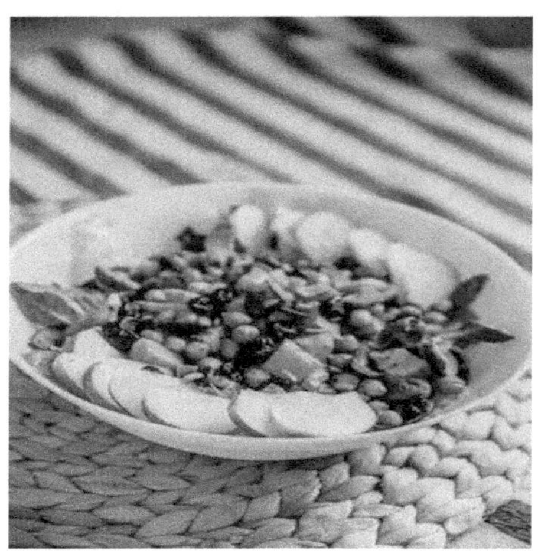

CHAPTER 5.

BEVERAGE OPTIONS FOR KIDNEY HEALTH:

Berry Blast Kidney-Friendly Smoothie

INGREDIENTS:

- 1 cup mixed berries (blueberries, strawberries, raspberries)
- 1 medium banana, peeled and sliced
- 1/2 cup low-fat or Greek yogurt
- 1/2 cup unsweetened almond milk
- 1 tablespoon chia seeds
- 1 tablespoon honey or maple syrup (optional, for sweetness)
- Ice cubes (optional)

INSTRUCTIONS:

- Blend together the mixed berries, sliced banana, low-fat or Greek yogurt, almond milk, and chia seeds in a blender.
- Add honey or maple syrup to the blender for a sweeter flavor.
- Blend until all of the ingredients are smooth and fully incorporated. If the smoothie is too thick, add additional almond milk to obtain the appropriate consistency.
- If you want your smoothie cold, mix in a handful of ice cubes until smooth.

Pour the kidney-friendly smoothie into a glass
and serve right away.

CHAPTER 6.

EATING OUT ON A RENAL DIET:

Grilled Lemon Herb Salmon with Quinoa and Steamed Vegetables

INGREDIENTS:

1. 4 salmon fillets (6 ounces each)
2. 1 lemon, sliced
3. 2 tablespoons olive oil
4. 2 teaspoons dried dill
5. 1 teaspoon dried thyme
6. 1 teaspoon garlic powder
7. Salt and pepper to taste

For the Quinoa:

1. 1 cup quinoa, rinsed
2. 2 cups low-sodium chicken or vegetable broth
3. 1/4 cup chopped fresh parsley

For the Steamed Vegetables:

1. 2 cups mixed vegetables (carrots, broccoli, and bell peppers work well)
2. 1 tablespoon olive oil
3. 1 teaspoon dried Italian herbs
4. Salt and pepper to taste

INSTRUCTIONS:

1. Preheat the grill to medium-high temperature.

2. To make the salmon marinade, combine the olive oil, dried dill, dried thyme, garlic powder, salt, and pepper in a small bowl.

3. Place the salmon fillets on a platter and brush with the marinade on both sides. Place a slice of lemon on top of each fillet.

4. Grill the salmon for 4-5 minutes per side, or until the fish readily flakes with a fork. Take care not to overcook.

5. Prepare the quinoa while the salmon is cooking. Combine the rinsed quinoa and chicken or vegetable broth in a medium saucepan. Bring to a boil, then lower to a low heat, cover, and cook for 15-20 minutes, or until the quinoa is tender and the liquid has been absorbed. With a

fork, fluff the quinoa and add in the parsley.

6. In a pan over medium heat, heat the olive oil for the steaming veggies. Combine the mixed veggies, dried Italian herbs, salt, and pepper in a mixing bowl. Cook until the veggies are soft but still crisp, about 5-7 minutes.

7. Serve the grilled lemon herb salmon over

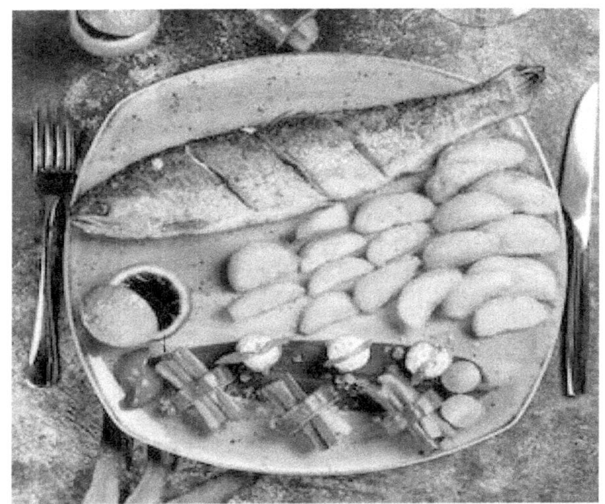

quinoa with steamed veggies on the side.

CHAPTER 7.

TIPS FOR LONG-TERM SUCCESS:

- Educate Yourself.

- Consult a Dietitian.

- Plan Balanced Meals.

- Mind Your Portions.

- Limit Processed Foods.

- Stay Hydrated

- Explore Kidney-Friendly Recipes

- Monitor Blood Pressure.

- Stay Positive and Persistent.

CONCLUSION

Additional Resources:

Enhancing Your Renal Diet Journey: A Comprehensive Resource Guide

Introduction:

Starting a renal diet demands not only commitment but also access to accurate information and assistance. To supplement your understanding of renal nutrition, we have compiled a list of supplementary materials ranging from meal planning to lifestyle changes. These materials attempt to provide you with the knowledge, recipes, and tools you need to effectively manage the complexities of a renal diet.

Renal Diet Recipes:

"Kidney Friendly Comfort Foods: A Collection of Low Potassium, Low Sodium, Kidney

Friendly Recipes" is written by Mathea Ford. This cookbook, which focuses on comfort meals, allows you to enjoy traditional cuisine while sticking to renal dietary restrictions. It features simple dishes that cater to a variety of taste preferences.

DaVita Community:

DaVita has a large online community with forums, blogs, and educational materials. This website, which focuses on kidney care, provides useful insights into maintaining renal health through shared experiences and professional assistance.

Websites for Education:

National Kidney Foundation (NKF): The NKF website is a comprehensive resource for kidney health information, including subjects such as food, drugs, and lifestyle. Learn about and manage your renal diet using instructional resources, articles, and tools.

The website of the American Association of Kidney Patients (AAKP) has a multitude of resources, including instructional materials, webinars, and articles. Investigate their Nutrition Counter feature, which provides nutritional information on a range of items to help with meal planning.

Podcasts:

"KidneyTalk" Podcast: KidneyTalk, produced by RSN, contains conversations with nephrology professionals covering all areas of kidney health, including food and nutrition. Stay informed and inspired on your renal diet journey by tuning in.

"The Renal Dietitian Podcast":

Hosted by a renal dietitian, this podcast looks into kidney health concerns, providing practical guidance and insights into efficiently managing a renal diet.